YOUR NEW BABY'S FIRST BIRTHDAY

AN OWNER'S 12-MONTH SERVICE GUIDE

BY MARTIN BAXENDALE

ISBN 0 9522032 2 7

Printed in Britain by Stoate and Bishop (Printers)
Ltd, Cheltenham and Gloucester

CONTENTS

INTRODUCTION   5

SERVICING AND REPAIRS   6

HEALTH AND SAFETY HAZARDS   15

NEW AND ADVANCED FEATURES,
FUNCTIONS AND OPERATING MODES   18

IMPROVED OPERATING SPECIFICATIONS
AND OPTIONAL ADD-ON ACCESSORIES   29

TECHNICAL INFORMATION   32

Also available in this series is:

Your New Baby - An Owner's Manual

An invaluable and hugely popular beginner's guide
to operating and maintaining a New Baby unit,
including a comprehensive introduction to the wide
range of useful and entertaining features and
functions readily available to even the most
inexperienced of owners and operators.
Guaranteed to ensure many years of trouble-
free operation (see legal note on following page).

"I don't know what I would have done without your
wonderful New Baby manual - I had no idea how to
work my New Baby properly and thought it might be
some kind of novel food-blender until I read your
marvellous handbook." (unsolicited letter from a
reader, Mr A.N. Idiot of Milton Keynes).

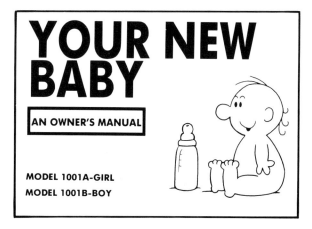

INTRODUCTION

In our basic handbook for beginners, Your New Baby - An Owner's Manual, we introduced proud new owners to the many standard features and functions, operating modes and day-to-day maintenance needs of the New Baby unit (model 1001A-GIRL or 1001B-BOY).

Now, as your New Baby reaches the end of its first year of operation, this comprehensive 12-month (or 2,000 nappy-changes) Service Guide is essential reading for the more experienced New Baby owner.

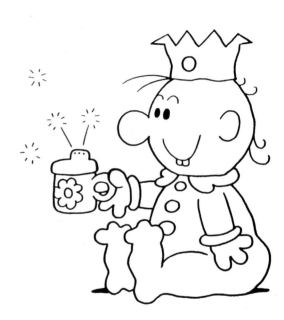

Crammed with valuable tips and hints to help you check the operating condition and performance of your one-year-old New Baby, it also provides a thorough up-date on the numerous <u>advanced</u> features, functions and modes that you will be sure to encounter (and come to love and enjoy) as you get to know your New Baby unit better with every passing month.

<u>Remember</u>, with careful and regular attention to recommended servicing and maintenance procedures your New Baby unit is guaranteed * to provide you with many years of trouble-free operation and countless hours of family fun and entertainment, whatever its age.

*LEGAL SMALL-PRINT:
Note; for the purposes of this guarantee, the phrase 'trouble-free' should in no way or manner be taken or construed to mean or suggest 'free from trouble'. Furthermore, it in no way infringes or affects your statutory right to be driven completely round the bend, weep and scream hysterically, run amuck with the bread-knife, and stake-out your darling little one-year-old on the nearest ant-hill.

SERVICING AND REPAIRS

FACTORY RECALL: Due to the considerable number of complaints received from New Baby owners about major design faults in their New Baby units, continuous and intolerable noise levels during operation, high running costs, and serious health and safety hazards to long-term New Baby operators, all New Baby units (Model 1001A-Girl and Model 1001B-Boy) are now subject to <u>AN URGENT FACTORY RECALL</u>.

Return your New Baby unit <u>immediately</u> for a complete overhaul to improved specifications. Due to back-logs in our workshops, this may take some weeks or even months, during which New Baby owners may wish to take a break, enjoy a holiday in the sun, just you, all alone, on your own.

We will return your New Baby unit to you free of all troublesome, annoying and niggling little drawbacks, easier to look after and keep clean, guaranteed absolutely trouble-free, cheaper to run, and much, much less noisy.....................bet we really had you going for a minute there! HA! HA! HA! HA! HA! HA!

PUBLISHER'S NOTE: We know that was a really evil trick, but we just couldn't resist it. Sorry.

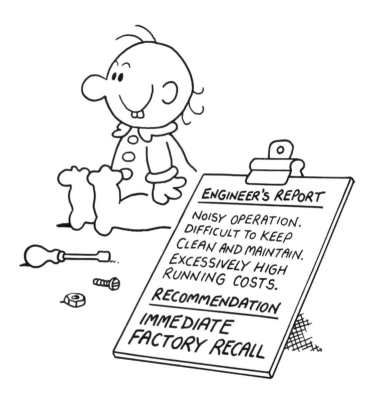

ENGINEER'S REPORT

NOISY OPERATION. DIFFICULT TO KEEP CLEAN AND MAINTAIN. EXCESSIVELY HIGH RUNNING COSTS.

RECOMMENDATION

IMMEDIATE FACTORY RECALL

COMMON FAULTS AND PROBLEM AREAS:

With older New Baby units, the commonest problems include: Excessively high operational noise levels (especially in teething mode), soft decorative outer casing very prone to damage from knocks, scrapes, scuffs, etc (particularly when unit is in self-propelling portable mode), ever-increasing running costs, and very real health and safety hazards to long-term New Baby owners and operators.

The following sections advise the advanced New Baby owner and operator on recommended service and repair procedures, and will help to ensure trouble-free operation whatever the age of your New Baby unit (or not, as the case may be).

ESSENTIAL SERVICING AND REPAIR MATERIALS:
For New Baby units of around 12-months old, the most useful servicing and repair materials include:

1) Teething granules. 2) Teething gel. 3) Arnica bump and bruise ointment 4) Hugs 5) Kisses

Be sure to have adequate supplies of these always available and apply liberally as required (see the following Service Record Chart).

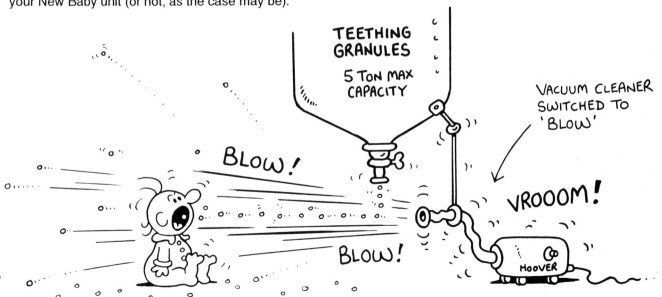

SERVICE RECORD CHART: To help you maintain a full and accurate service history for your New Baby unit, please complete the following Service Record Chart, ticking and dating the boxes as and when the appropriate service levels have been reached.

SERVICING LEVEL	TICK	DATE
First container of teething granules used up		
2nd " " " " " "		
First hundredweight sack of granules bought		
First bulk lorryload of granules delivered		
First tube of teething gel used up		
2nd " " " " " "		
3rd " " " " " "		
Teething gel drip-feed fitted to New Baby		
First tube of bump ointment used up		
2nd " " " " " "		
3rd " " " " " "		
The first time you find that you're getting through a 50-gallon drum a day		

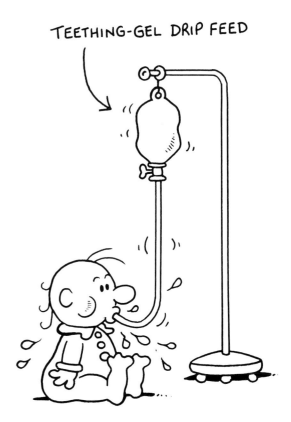

TEETHING-GEL DRIP FEED

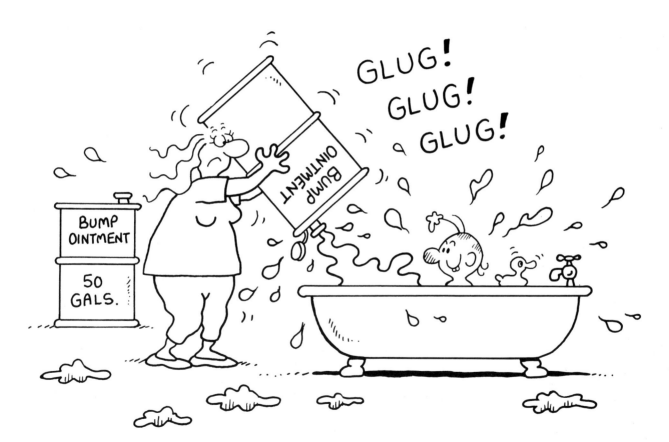

EMERGENCY REPAIR WORKSHOPS:

You're likely to need to rush your New Baby unit to an emergency repair workshop more than once in its earliest years; usually for specialist attention to unsightly knocks, scrapes, scuffs, minor burns, etc, spoiling the appearance of the New Baby unit's soft decorative outer casing.

To avoid panic, we strongly recommend that you locate in advance your nearest authorised emergency repair and servicing centre, and carefully memorise the shortest available route.

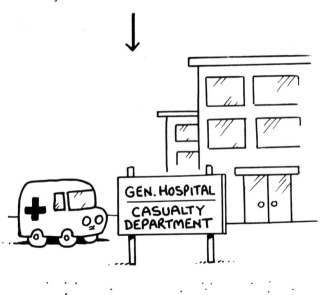

DAMAGE TO DECORATIVE SOFT OUTER CASING OF NEW BABY UNIT:

This is one of the commonest servicing and repair problems faced by owners and operators of older New Baby units, especially when the unit starts operating in self-propelled portable mode.

Damage can take numerous forms, as can be seen from the accompanying illustrations. In most cases, applying the basic servicing lubricants, Arnica bump ointment, Hugs, and Kisses, will produce a perfectly adequate repair.

In case of more serious damage, or if at all concerned about the adequacy of your own repair procedures, see section on Emergency Repair Workshops.

NOTE: The good news is that your New Baby unit carries a full <u>Bodywork Lifetime Rust-Proof Guarantee</u> courtesy of the manufacturers and completely free of charge.

WARNING: No matter how tatty your New Baby unit's decorative outer casing may start to look (ingrained food residues, bumps, scratches, etc) <u>under no circumstances</u> attempt a re-spray job. Most blemishes can (eventually) be removed by vigorous cleaning with soapy water or applications of the recommended service/repair materials.

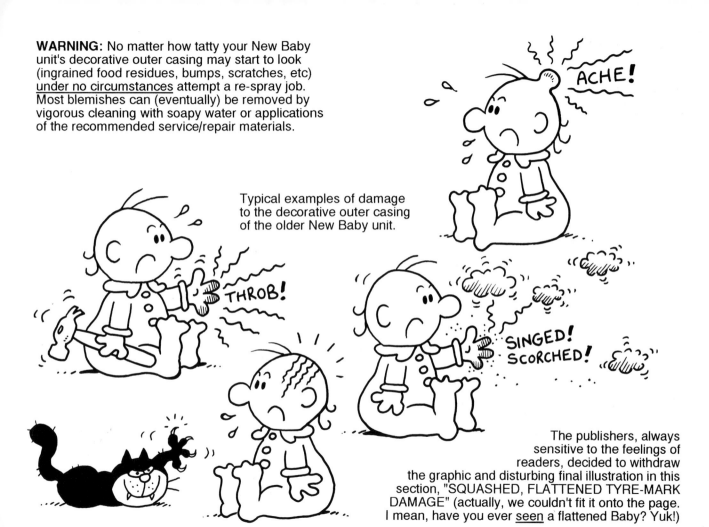

ACHE!

Typical examples of damage to the decorative outer casing of the older New Baby unit.

THROB!

SINGED!
SCORCHED!

The publishers, always sensitive to the feelings of readers, decided to withdraw the graphic and disturbing final illustration in this section, "SQUASHED, FLATTENED TYRE-MARK DAMAGE" (actually, we couldn't fit it onto the page. I mean, have you ever <u>seen</u> a flattened Baby? Yuk!)

NOISY OPERATION: Noise levels are likely to be highest and most ear-piercing in the following operating modes: Teething mode; Whingeing mode; Whining mode; Tantrum mode, etc. In most of these operating modes, excessive noise levels are normally only a temporary problem, usually ending when your New Baby unit changes from one mode to another.

Your New Baby may also emit extremely high noise levels temporarily when switching from Awake mode to Sleep mode. This is quite normal and you should try to ignore it. Note: Despite appearances, your New Baby unit is <u>not</u> about to explode.....although it would like you to think that it is. (See also 'Bedtime infra-red movement detector and alarm function' in chapter on new and advanced features and functions).

If excessively high operating noise levels prove to be a long-term, virtually continuous nuisance then your New Baby unit is probably in Teething mode, and you have our deepest sympathy . In addition to advice given earlier (see section on servicing materials and service record chart) attaching a Teething-comforter add-on accessory to your New Baby unit may help to reduce operational noise levels (more technically speaking, give it something to chew on; a teething ring, rubber dog's bone, Dad's finger, tractor tyre...)

You may also experience noisy operation of your New Baby unit immediately following damage to its soft decorative casing (see earlier section in this chapter). In this event, quickly apply generous quantities of the basic servicing and repair materials (Bump-ointment, Hugs, and Kisses) until noise levels are back to normal.

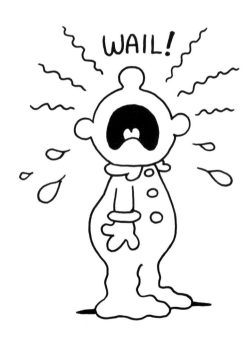

WAIL!

DIRECTIONAL GUIDANCE SYSTEM
MALFUNCTION: Due to a basic design fault, your New Baby unit's directional guidance system is prone to malfunctioning, so that when in self-propelling portable mode, it will inevitably at some point give a big grin, do a U-turn and shoot off in exactly the opposite direction to where you want it to go.

The recommended sequence of correctional procedures is as follows: 1) Yell 2) Scream 3) Grab 4) Drag. (See also section on Noisy Operation, and section on Walking Reins Steering Accessory under IMPROVED OPERATING SPECIFICATIONS AND OPTIONAL ADD-ON ACCESSORIES).

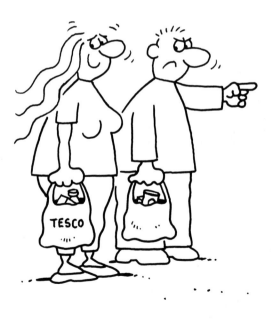

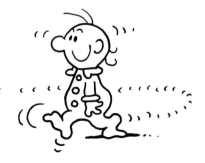

FAULTY ON/OFF SWITCH: Another common problem caused by an uncorrectable design fault. Sorry. See 'Switching from Awake mode to Asleep mode' in earlier section on Noisy operation.

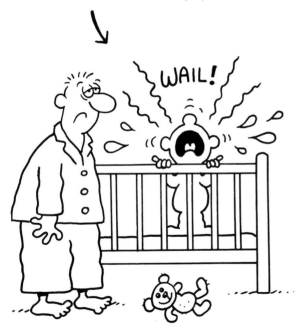

HIGH RUNNING-COSTS: We regret that the older your New Baby unit gets the higher the running costs will inevitably become.

And we're not talking the occasional half-litre of oil and a new spark-plug here. We are talking serious dosh. We are talking a new clothes size every 3-months, a new pair of shoes a week, school clothes, fashion clothes, jeans, trainers, Cindy dolls, Barbie dolls, skateboards, CDs, tapes, computer games, school trips, ridiculous trendy haircuts, pocket money.....

Sorry, but didn't anyone tell you? It's not like it wasn't mentioned in all the advertising, you know (well okay, so maybe it wasn't).

HEALTH AND SAFETY HAZARDS

Unfortunately, due to countless design flaws and programming errors, your average New Baby unit constitutes a serious health and safety hazard to long-term owners and operators.

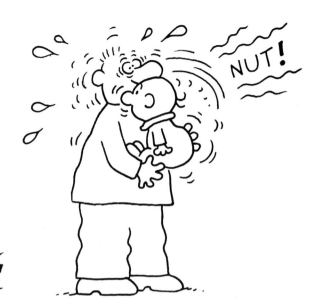

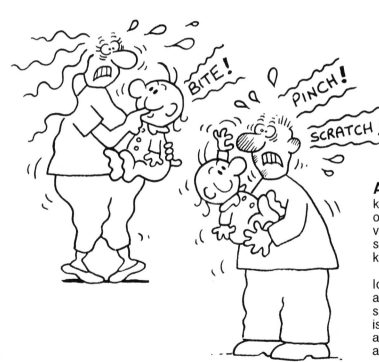

ACCIDENTAL INJURY: Firstly, take care to keep your fingers, nose, eyes, ears, mouth, and all other body-parts well clear of your New Baby unit's various dangerously sharp, nastily biting, viciously scratching, sneakily pinching, scratching, gouging, kicking, hitting and head-butting bits.

Ideally, your New Baby unit's new teeth, fingernails and rock-hard head should be fitted with operator safety-guards at all times. But installation of these is unfortunately not covered by the Health and Safety at Work Act. It is also likely to attract the unwelcome attention of the local social services and the RSPCC.

REPETITIVE STRAIN INJURY is yet another health hazard to the long-term New Baby unit operator. The overall repetitive strain of coping with a New Baby unit day after day, week after week, year after year, can constitute a very real mental health hazard (or, to put it more technically, it can do your head in).

Physically, the repetitive strain of repeatedly picking-up-and-carrying your New Baby unit as it gets older can cause severe medical problems; as can the repetitive strain of constant nappy-changing, repeated putting-back-down-in-the-cot at bedtime, continually picking-up teddies, toys, drink beakers, etc. thrown from prams, high-chairs and cots, etc, etc, etc, etc.

The best way to avoid repetitive strain injury when operating your New Baby unit for prolonged periods is to take plenty of breaks away from the unit at regular intervals throughout the working day, doing other things (even if it's only a coffee break or locking yourself in the loo for five minute's peace and quiet).

Job-sharing can also help, if you have a partner who will periodically take over operation of the New Baby unit, sharing operational tasks and reducing the stress and strain of continual single-operator running of the unit.

No, don't laugh. This is serious.

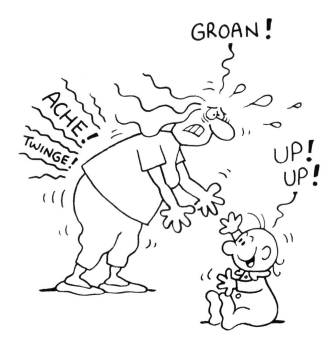

DANGER OF INFECTION: You will probably also have noticed by now your New Baby unit's infallible ability to catch and pass on to you every sniffle, cold, tummy bug, mystery virus, etc that is going around; and even a few that <u>aren't</u> going around.

Indeed, our research department are currently working on the theory that the average New Baby unit is actually a highly efficient miniature <u>biological warfare facility</u> producing more bugs than Porton Down, and of potential military interest to various aggressive small countries who can't afford a nuclear weapons programme.

Moves are believed to be under discussion at the highest international levels to make all New Baby units worldwide subject to regular compulsory inspections by United Nations biological warfare investigation teams.

In the meantime, we strongly recommend the use of surgical gloves, masks, breathing apparatus, lead-lined suits, remote-control arms, and any other precautions you can think of or afford, whenever you have to handle a New Baby unit with the slightest hint of a sniffle, a runny bottom half or a pukey top half.

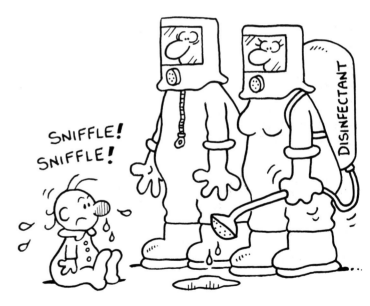

NEW AND ADVANCED FEATURES, FUNCTIONS AND OPERATING MODES

You should have discovered by now that your New Baby unit's capacity for displaying a wide range of operating modes, features and functions rapidly increases with time.

The more experienced New Baby unit owner/operator will, by the end of the first 12-months or 2,000 nappy-changes service period, be discovering exciting, useful and entertaining new features and functions almost every week.

Here are just a few of those you're most likely to encounter during normal day-to-day running of the unit. Enjoy.

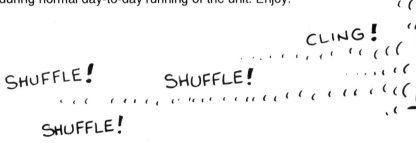
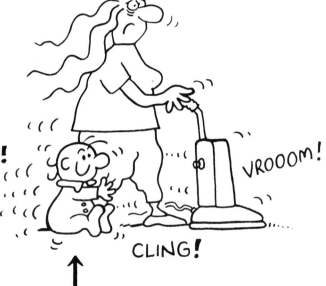

BALL-AND-CHAIN MODE: You will find that your New Baby unit is most likely to switch into this operating mode just when you need to do something that involves a lot of walking around; hoovering, going out to hang up the washing, nipping upstairs to the loo, walking to the shops, etc. Very helpful.

SELF-PROPELLING PORTABLE MODE

This operates in various sub-modes, including:

CRAWLING-AND-BUMPING-INTO-THINGS
CRAWLING-AND-FALLING-DOWNSTAIRS
WALKING-AND-BUMPING-INTO-THINGS
WALKING-AND-TRIPPING-UP
RUNNING-AND-FALLING-OVER
ESCAPING

See also section on Steering Reins Accessory, under OPTIONAL ADD-ON ACCESSORIES, Directional Guidance System Malfunction under SERVICING AND REPAIRS, and section on Portability under UP-RATED PERFORMANCE SPECIFICATIONS.

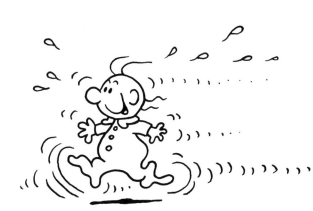

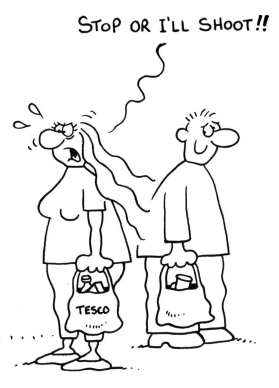

STOP OR I'LL SHOOT!!

CARRY MODE: This is very similar in effect to Ball-And-Chain Mode and tends to switch into operation in pretty much the same circumstances; but especially if you are already carrying great piles of heavy shopping bags, washing, etc. Even more helpful.

See also Repetitive Strain Injury, under HEALTH AND SAFETY HAZARDS.

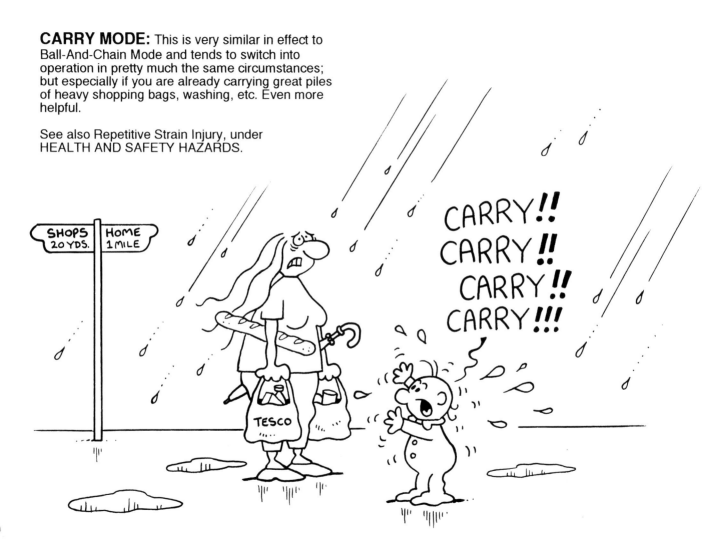

TELEPHONE MODEM FUNCTION: Your New Baby unit should, by the end of its first 12 months of operation, have fully developed the capability to act as an independent telephone modem, freely interfacing with the local, national and international telephone systems whenever you turn your back for five minutes.

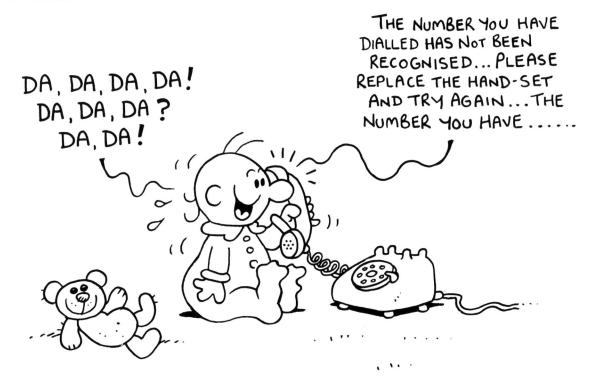

YOUR NEW BABY AS AN AUTOMATIC DISPOSAL UNIT:

This useful feature completely frees you from the tiresome effort of having to dispose of unwanted objects such as jewellery, purses, wallets, watches, cutlery, books, ornaments, small domestic pets, etc, etc.

Your New Baby unit will simply and neatly dispose of them for you, whenever you aren't looking, into the kitchen rubbish bin, down the toilet, under the settee, behind the radiators, and a thousand other places where you'll never see or find them again.

No, please don't thank us. It's all part of the service.

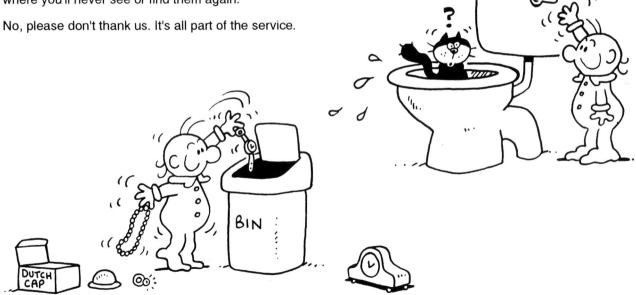

CUPBOARD-OPENING-AND-EMPTYING
FUNCTION: A highly entertaining feature of the older New Baby unit, usually combined with the equally enjoyable Bashing-Pan-Lids-Together function. An exciting game-playing operating mode, guaranteed to relax even the most stressed-out of New Baby unit owner/operators. Compete with your New Baby unit for the highest cupboard door-slamming and finger-trapping score (Sorry! Your New Baby unit always wins!)

Note: Drawer-Opening-And-Emptying is a similarly exciting game-playing mode. This time, you are competing to see if you can re-fold and put back your knickers, bras, boxer shorts, socks, etc. as fast as your New Baby unit throws them out! Non-stop thrills and spills, and plenty of action!

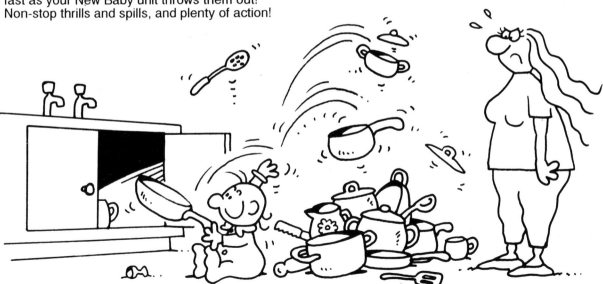

BEDTIME INFRA-RED MOVEMENT DETECTOR AND ALARM FUNCTION

To test the operation of this interesting feature, first put your New Baby unit down in its night-time storage facility (cot or bed).

When the unit is soundly in Sleep mode and snoring, test by attempting to move v-e-r-y s-l-o-w-l-y and silently in pitch darkness away from the cot/bed towards the door. If this function is operating correctly, your New Baby unit should emit an ear-piercing alarm shriek before you can move more than an inch in the direction of the door.

See also Noisy Operation section under SERVICING AND REPAIRS.

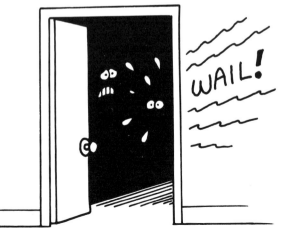

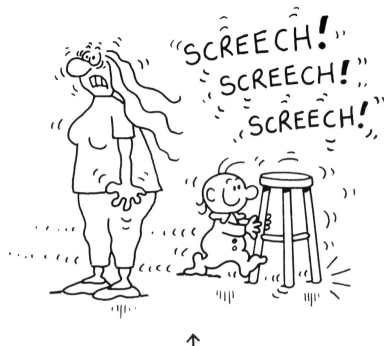

FURNITURE RE-ARRANGING MODE

Never again worry about how best to arrange your furniture; leave it all to your New Baby unit's in-built interior design programming. Will produce fantastic interior decor effects like you've never dreamed of; all your furniture heaped decoratively in one corner, all your chairs and stools trendily upside-down, rugs rolled-up and artistically arranged in the fireplace, table cloths tastefully draped over domestic pets, etc., etc.

DOOR-SLAMMING MODE: An extremely useful feature. Never again will you need to shut a door behind you. Simply leave it to your New Baby unit. Indeed, eventually it will be impossible to leave any door in the house open for more than a few seconds before your New Baby unit spots it and closes it for you.

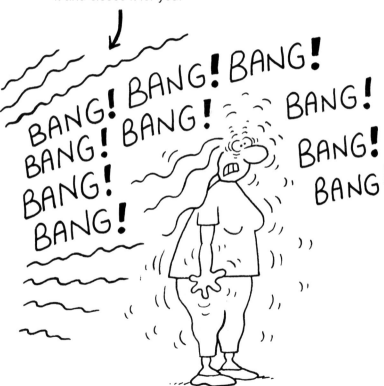

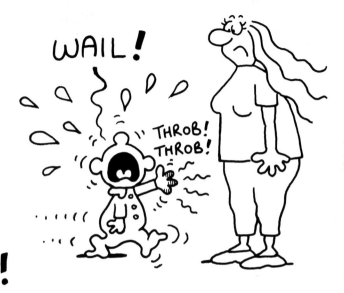

Unfortunately, this operating feature will often switch automatically into <u>Repeat</u> Door-Slamming Mode, which can prove even more annoying. Sorry. Small programming error.

It may also lead to accidental damage to your New Baby unit's soft decorative outer casing in the fingers area (see SERVICING AND REPAIRS).

Applies equally to cupboard doors (see also Cupboard-Opening-And-Emptying Function).

SELF-PLUGGING-IN FUNCTION: You may find that your New Baby unit repeatedly spends a great deal of operating time attempting to initiate this function and connect itself to your household electrical supply.

We strongly recommend that you discourage these attempts, as a domestic electrical supply is a highly unsuitable power-source on which to run a New Baby unit and can cause irreparable damage. Electrical socket guards are also readily available from many high-street shops and can be easily fitted for peace of mind.

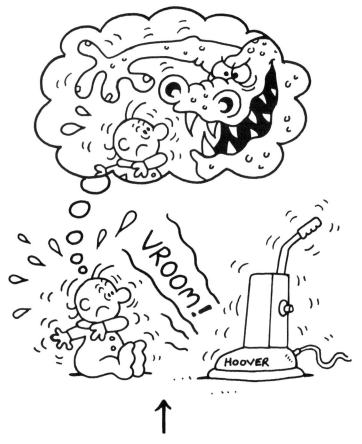

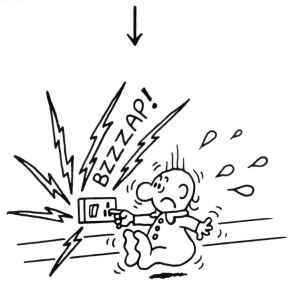

HOOVER-MONSTER PARANOIA MODE

No, we shouldn't laugh. It's not funny. The poor little thing. No, stop it. Really, it isn't funny....don't go and switch the hoover on........

26

PLAY MODE: On balance, we'd probably say that it's best <u>not</u> to encourage operation of Play Mode, as the little buggers will only want to do it on your bed at five in the morning, when even the sparrows are still snoring and you want another couple of hours with your head under the duvet.

But then we'd have those interfering New Baby unit educational psychology nerds from our research and development department on our backs, so........do encourage operation of Play Mode in your New Baby unit at all times, as it is an essential aid to the development of your New Baby's future programming and advanced operating functions. Honest.

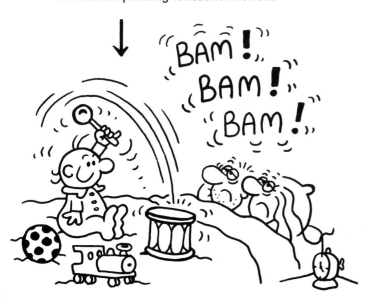

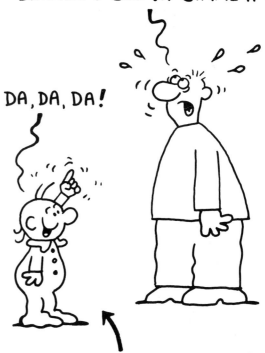

AIMLESS POINTING FUNCTION: A particularly puzzling and annoying New Baby unit function with no purpose that our engineers can discover. Probably best to just ignore it, otherwise it'll drive you mad.

BONK-BUSTING MODE: An <u>extremely</u> annoying feature of the older New Baby unit, and one which our frustrated research department have been working night and day to eradicate, without success.

Basically, it's the average older New Baby unit's uncanny ability to sense when joint owner/operators Mummy and Daddy fancy a quick bit of naughties; to immediately interrupt and/or shove itself between them, and steadfastly refuse to be distracted by offers of other activities no matter how tempting or normally prohibited; such as being given the telephone to play with, Mummy's jewellery, Daddy's credit cards, small and vulnerable domestic pets, or assorted electrical appliances and unguarded sockets.

We're still working on it. There has to be an answer. Trust us. We'll find it. We hope. Oh God, we do hope so.

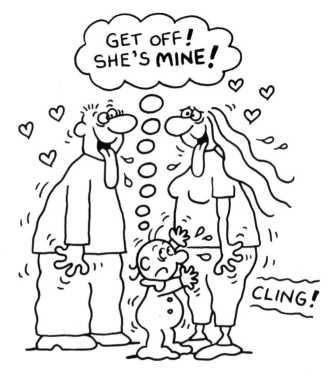

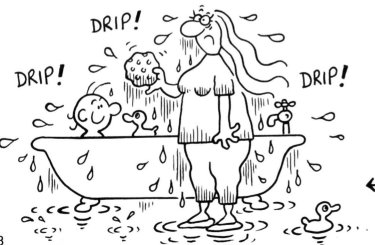

BATHROOM-FLOODING FUNCTION

This operating mode frequently switches into automatic operation whenever you attempt to clean the decorative outer casing of older New Baby units, making an umbrella and wellies essential bath-time wear for the average owner/operator.

IMPROVED OPERATING SPECIFICATIONS AND OPTIONAL ADD-ON ACCESSORIES

Various functions and modes of your New Baby unit are automatically up-graded to higher specifications as the unit's accumulated operating time increases over the months and years.

There are also one or two useful add-on accessories for the older New Baby unit which will help to further improve and up-grade performance in some of the more crucial operating functions.

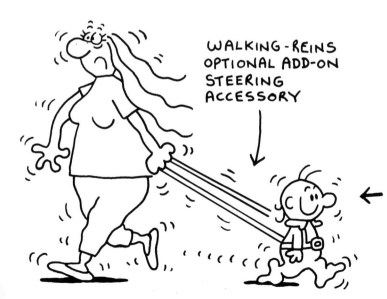

WALKING-REINS OPTIONAL ADD-ON STEERING ACCESSORY

PORTABILITY: Your New Baby unit was originally advertised as a "fully portable lap-size model" (see Your New Baby - An Owner's Manual, also published in this series).

With time and experience, your New Baby unit should prove even <u>more</u> portable (if not exactly remaining lap-size for ever); indeed, with time, the unit should develop an up-graded Self-Propelling Portable Mode (see NEW AND ADVANCED FEATURES, FUNCTIONS AND OPERATING MODES).

This is an extremely useful feature but, unfortunately, not entirely reliable. It tends to suddenly switch off without warning and revert to <u>Carry Mode</u> over distances of more than a few yards. The Directional Guidance System is also prone to malfunctioning in Self-Propelling Mode, so that your New Baby unit will tend to constantly wander off in any direction but the one you want it to go in.

Something that you may or may not find helpful is the optional add-on Walking-Reins Steering Accessory. The one major draw-back with this is that most people completely misunderstand its purpose and function. Far from being an aid to steering your New Baby unit, the Walking-Reins Accessory is in fact of immense help to your New Baby unit in steering <u>you</u> in the direction <u>he/she</u> wants to go. An easy mistake to make, but we thought we'd better point it out to avoid further confusion and disappointment.

OVERFLOW/WASTE-DISPOSAL FUNCTION:

New Baby unit running costs and owner/operator labour can be drastically reduced by replacing the earlier disposable/washable Nappy Waste-Disposal Add-On Unit with the up-graded <u>Potty</u> unit.

Sounds easy, doesn't it. The trouble is that <u>fitting</u> the up-graded Potty Overflow/Waste-Disposal <u>Unit</u> is not exactly easy. The problem is getting it to stay connected to the New Baby unit long enough for the overflow/waste-disposal function to be completed (or even started).

<u>WARNING</u>: Under no circumstances can we recommend the use of <u>super-glue</u> or a <u>staple-gun</u> in attempting to fix the advanced Potty Overflow/Waste-Disposal Unit to your New Baby (however much we might sympathise with your predicament). You could always try cellotape or parcel-tape. By the way, we've tried Blu-Tack and it's useless.

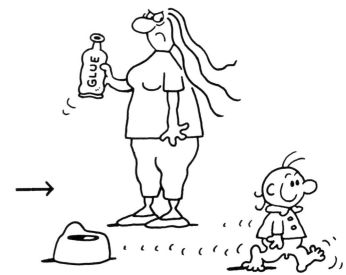

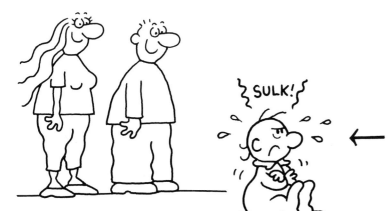

TANTRUM MODE: This is an unfortunate but inevitable up-grade on your New Baby unit's earlier <u>Whingeing Mode</u>. To compare the two is like comparing a mild Earth-tremor to a full-scale volcanic eruption complete with boiling lava-flows, belching poisonous gases and coastal tidal-waves.

SULKING MODE: A new feature of the older New Baby unit, usually following closely after operation of <u>Tantrum Mode</u>. Try not to laugh. Your New Baby is really pissed off with you and is trying to demonstrate it.....no matter how ridiculous he/she may look.